The 28 Day Plan

FLAT STOMACH

Christine Green

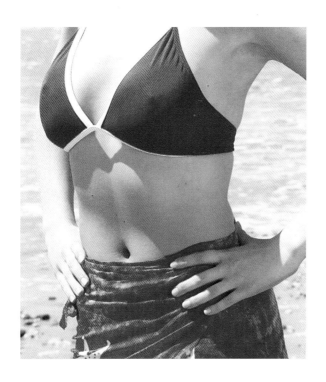

p

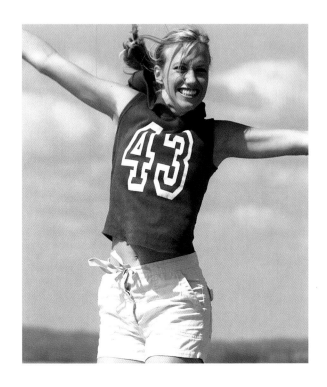

This is a Parragon Publishing Book

First published by Parragon 2002

Parragon Publishing
Queen Street House
4 Queen Street
Bath BA1 1HE, UK

Copyright © Parragon 2002

Designed, produced and packaged by
Stonecastle Graphics Limited

Text by Christine Green
Edited by Gillian Haslam
Designed by Sue Pressley and Paul Turner
Commissioned photography by Roddy Paine

ISBN 0-75256-802-7

Printed in China

Disclaimer

The exercises and advice detailed in this book
assume that you are a normally healthy adult.
Therefore the author, publishers, their servants or
agents cannot accept responsibility for loss or
damage suffered by individuals as a result of
following advice or attempting an exercise or
treatment referred to in this book. It is strongly
recommended that individuals intending to
undertake an exercise program and any change
of diet do so following consultation with their
medical practitioner.

Contents

You Can Have a Flat Stomach

Have you striven for years to attain a well-toned lean stomach; have you tried every diet imaginable; stuck rigidly to a daily ritual of sit-ups and even contemplated spending your savings on liposuction, all for the sake of having a flat stomach?

Forget all that and enroll yourself on this 28-day program which will guarantee you trim and well-toned abdominal muscles and a stomach to be proud of. And with the money you have saved by not choosing liposuction, treat yourself to a new outfit to show off your flat stomach.

Reasons for a flabby stomach

Why is it that some people who have never eaten a crispbread in their life, never ventured into a gym, and for whom "healthy" eating is a dirty word still have washboard-like stomachs to die for? Is genetics to blame, the after-effects of childbirth, bad eating habits, a sedentary lifestyle, even bad posture? All are possibilities but there are also several other reasons including:

- Age
- Beer belly
- Lack of exercise
- Motherhood
- Stress
- The monthly cycle
- Trapped wind

Lack of exercise

If you plan to follow this 28-day program, you must give up feeble excuses such as you haven't time, you are too busy, or that you have something better to do – the only way to deal with excess flab around the middle is a combined program of exercise and healthy eating.

Extra flesh gained around the abdominal area is difficult to move because, once those fat cells have formed, although they may shrink in size they are constantly lying in wait, ready to pounce in response to a moment's lapse. If you don't work the muscles, they will turn flabby, but once they are regularly exercised, toned, and strengthened, they respond in no time at all.

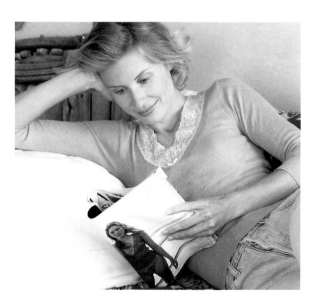

Your age

It is a pity that so much attention nowadays is focused upon the way a woman looks and the changes caused by aging, especially when you are over 30.

In truth this is the age when a woman's metabolism naturally slows down, because the body has reached a turning point when nature is equipping it with extra baggage, generally in the shape of excess flesh around the waist, thighs, and upper arms. The only remedy is to accept these changes gracefully, but at the same time to fight back.

By all means enjoy the occasional cream cake but make sure it is just "occasional." Experts recommend that the only way to keep your shape in trim is to reduce your intake of calories and to increase the amount of exercise you take. And that's what this 28-day program is all about.

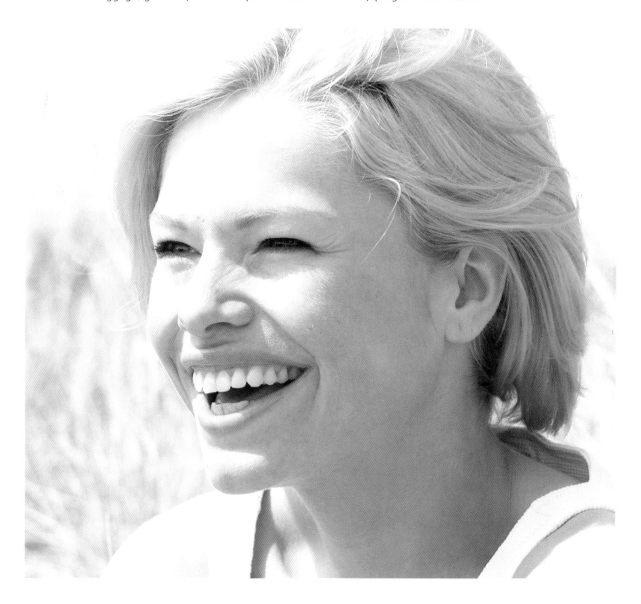

Bloating

The "time of the month" plays havoc not only with emotions but also body shape, sometimes making you feel that you look like a beached whale! The hormone progesterone is the guilty party. Generally a week before the onset of your period, the body begins to produce extra progesterone (the hormone responsible for causing fluid retention) in preparation for an egg to be fertilized. Naturally this fluid manifests itself around the stomach. Once the "all-clear" signal is heard and the body knows that it is not pregnant, progesterone levels drop to their normal level, excess fluid is released through your urine, and the stomach returns to its normal shape.

It is during this difficult build-up period that your mind often plays tricks on you. The raised levels of progesterone can affect one's mood and body image, so although rationally you know you aren't any fatter, you still feel that you are.

Trapped wind

The body is an amazing organism but there are times when it refuses to accept quietly the foods it is being fed and reacts in unpredictable ways. Many find complex sugar foods, such as fruit, vegetables, and beans, are difficult to digest and the result is intestinal gas that can give the stomach a rather bloated appearance and an uncomfortable feeling of fullness.

The most effective way to deal with this is to monitor your diet and eliminate those foods which are responsible.

Stress

Whenever you are worried or under stress, the body reacts. Some people find that the stomach is particularly affected when it is suddenly bombarded with large amounts of the stress hormone cortisol.

Because the stomach area has more receptors than any other part of the body, the hormone is automatically pumped into the fat cells lying around the waist where it settles.

In order to deal with stress and to reduce the effect it has on your stomach, there are several positive things you can do:

- Learn to relax
- Take regular exercise
- Practice deep breathing
- Have a good laugh
- If you drink or smoke, cut down

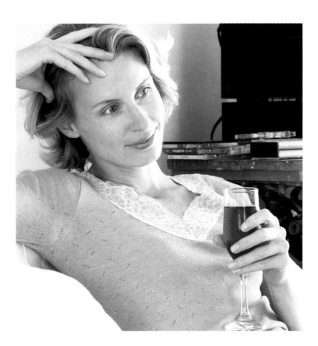

Beer Belly

Beer is not the only culprit; in fact any alcoholic drink can increase the size of the stomach simply because every gram of alcohol contains seven calories, almost twice as many per gram of most other carbohydrates or protein. So if you know that alcohol is the cause of your flabby stomach, there is only one answer: give up drinking the stuff!

Why toned muscles look so much better

Looking good and feeling good go hand in hand and the fact that you are conscious of your flabby stomach muscles will do little to boost your self-confidence and make you feel good about yourself. So time invested in dealing with the problem will change your whole outlook on life:

✓ You will look good in whatever clothes you wear

✓ Your confidence in yourself will soar

✓ Your posture will be improved

✓ You will not suffer back discomfort

By the end of the 28 days

If you have decided to undertake this program, rest assured that you will not regret it. Just don't become too obsessive about what you eat, or about the amount of exercise you try to do. Set yourself realistic targets, ones that you know you can achieve. Make up a chart and monitor your daily progress, marking down how many sit-ups or stomach exercises you managed on a particular day and then try increasing them the following day, but do it gradually. Keep reminding yourself why you are doing it.

Read these six motivational sentences each time you feel your willpower sagging:

I will keep focused, and by the end of these 28 days I will:

- **Feel healthier**
- **Feel more confident**
- **Feel much better about how I look in snug-fitting clothes**
- **Will want to wear short cropped tops**
- **Will not have a bad back**
- **My posture will be improved**

By the end of the program, with perseverance and dedication, you will have achieved every one of them.

No more excuses about starting tomorrow or next week, there is no time like today! So start planning now and let's get working toward your dream of achieving perfect flat abs.

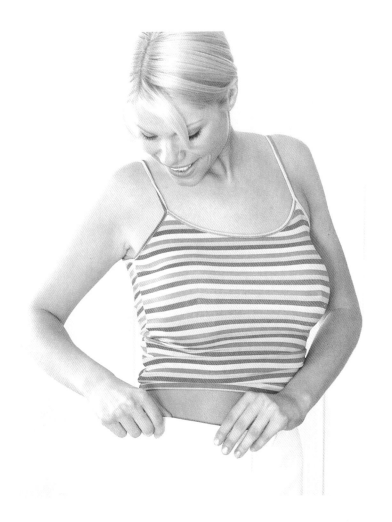

Learning To Exercise

A large part of this program deals with exercise and in particular how to tone the abdominal muscles that work in conjunction with the back muscles to help maintain good posture. But sometimes all the hard work can come to nothing because it is not fully understood how the abdominal muscles work.

Stomach muscles

Before you start to exercise your abdominal muscles, it is important to understand how they work.

Basically the stomach area is made up of four main abdominal muscles:

Internal and external obliques

Two diagonal lengths of muscle called the external and internal obliques run across the front of the ribs and around to the spine. Their primary function is to help the torso when twisting, bending from side to side, and also to maintain its stability

Tranversus abdominis (deep)

Running horizontally from the lower ribs to the spine, this group of muscles hold and maintain the shape of the organs within the abdomen. Each time we hold our stomachs in, these are the muscles which are working.

Rectus abdominis (front)

A muscle that runs vertically from the sternum to the pubic bone – its main role is to help move the torso from a lying position to an upright one. Problems occur as weight is put on around the midsection and

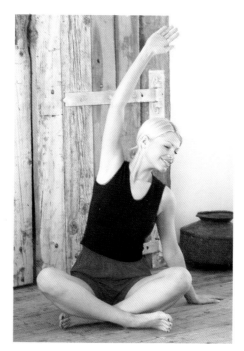

the muscles are engulfed beneath it and become unable to retain their former defined shape.

As more weight settles, then it doesn't matter if you wear a girdle or hold your stomach in all day, it will not make any difference. The fat is there to stay unless you decide to do something about it – and that means exercise. Without regular exercise, the muscles will begin to weaken and you will find yourself with a flabby stomach.

When to exercise

Many experts recommend exercising first thing in the morning but it really depends on individual preference.

If, for example, you are in full-time employment, you may find yourself having to exercise in the morning or evening, either before you leave for work or after you return home. If you have young children, you may well choose to exercise when they are at school or playgroup. The most important thing is to choose a time which is convenient for you and with which you feel comfortable.

How to begin exercising

Providing you are under 35 and in good health, there is little reason to see a doctor before embarking on an exercise program. However, if you have recently given birth or been inactive for several years, then you should, for your own safety, consider making an appointment to see your doctor first.

If you suffer from any of these medical conditions, you should definitely seek medical advice:

- Arthritis or other bone problems
- Extreme breathlessness after mild exertion
- Family history of early stroke or heart attacks
- Frequent dizzy spells
- Heart trouble
- High blood pressure
- Other known or suspected disease
- Severe muscular, ligament, or tendon problems

Basic warm-up movements

Loosening up the body before exercising is important because it prepares the muscles and joints for the workout and also increases the heart rate causing the blood to pump faster around the body. Consequently the harder the muscles work, the more beneficial the exercise will be. There are lots of warm-up exercises to choose from but basically they should be a blend of rhythmic stretching so that all parts of the body are limbered up and ready to go.

Shoulders To loosen up tense shoulder and neck

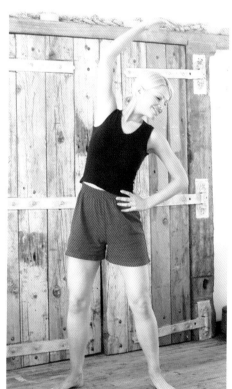

muscles, stand with your feet slightly apart, then roll the left shoulder backward ten times. Repeat with the right shoulder, at the same time shifting your weight from the left foot to the right foot.

Arms and knees This is a great one for overall posture. Stand up straight, stomach tucked in, then swing both arms up and then swing them down, bending the knees as you bring the arms down in a gentle smooth action. Repeat 15 times.

Side to side With your feet evenly spaced apart, knees gently bent and hands firmly on the hips, very slowly lean over to one side stretching the arm out at the same time as far as you can. Return to a standing position and stretch to the other side. Repeat four stretches on each side.

Waisting time This is good for the spine and waist. With your feet slightly parted, knees gently bent, hips facing forward, raise the arms nearly to shoulder level and, taking it easy, twist the body from side to side. Do four twists each side.

Stretching Sitting on the floor cross-legged, place one hand slightly behind you, then bring the other arm up and, with the palm facing outward, stretch up as far as you are able. Hold for the count of ten, bring the arm back down and repeat with the other arm.

Body stretch This is a pleasant exercise. Simply lie on your back and stretch your arms and legs as far as possible. Hold for five seconds and then relax.

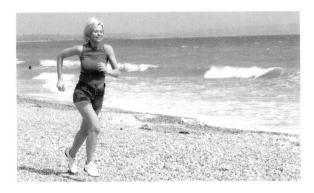

Types of Exercise

There are two main types of exercise that will help you to attain a flat stomach. One is aerobic exercise and the other is toning or strengthening work. Both are important.

Aerobic exercises

These exercises help to burn fat and involve any form of activity that makes you feel a little out of breath. They include:

- Cycling
- Jogging
- Power walking
- Running
- Skipping
- Swimming

Toning or strengthening exercises

These exercises build up specific muscle groups and, in doing so, increase the rate at which calories are used up.

Some exercises to try

There are many different toning and strengthening exercises which are perfect for getting to work on the abdominals. Ideally you should try doing each of these exercises slowly and carefully, concentrating on the areas of the body on which you are working. Start by doing 5–10 minutes each day, and aim to build up to about 20. You will find a workout mat very useful for the floor exercises.

Crunch

The basic exercise for strengthening and toning the upper abdominals.

1. Lie with your back flat on the floor, knees bent and feet spaced shoulder-width apart.

2. Place your hands behind your ears but do not hold on to your head or neck.

3. Now for the difficult part. Keeping your eyes focused directly on the ceiling and your elbows wide apart, slowly raise your shoulders off the ground, pulling in the stomach muscles as you do so. Do not try to raise more than your shoulders off the floor.

4. Then slowly lower the shoulders back to the floor, remembering to exhale as you come up and inhale as you lower down again.

5. At this stage don't push yourself and risk putting undue strain on your back. It isn't the quantity of crunches that matters, it's the quality.

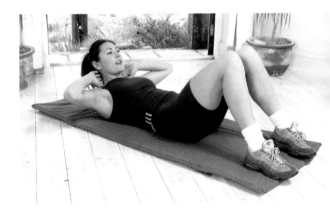

Ready to crunch

Here is a handy tip if you find ab crunches rather difficult: spend 3 minutes lying flat on your back pressing your spine into the floor and holding your stomach muscles tight for a count of ten. Twenty a day should enable you to progress to trying a few crunches after a few days.

Full sit-ups

1. Lie on the floor in the same position as for the crunch with your hands gently resting behind your ears.

2. Now pull your whole body up as far as you can, remembering to exhale as you rise up and keeping your feet flat on the ground. The aim is to sit upright, but very few people manage this in the beginning, so don't worry too much if you cannot do it. Just go as far as you can without feeling any undue strain on your back.

3. Slowly roll back down to the floor, remembering to inhale.

4. Then relax for a moment, gather your energy and have another try.

Isometric abdominal curl

An ideal exercise for strengthening all the abdominal muscles.

1. Lie flat on your back, hands gently placed behind the ears.

2. Place your feet flat on the floor, with the heels pulled up close to your buttocks.

3. Tighten your abdominal muscles and at the same time push your lower back down into the floor.

4. With your back now firmly on the ground, lift your feet just a couple of inches up off the floor, hold for ten seconds.

5. Then slowly release, rest and repeat.

Cooling down

Just as you need to prepare the body for exercising with warming-up exercises, you also need to cool it down after you have finished. After all, your body has been through quite an ordeal! You will find lots of different warming-up and cooling-down exercises in various books but here are a few of my favorites for you to try.

Tips for sit-ups

As with most forms of exercise it is important to get the maximum benefit out of each. Many people fail to do sit-ups correctly so here are a few important pointers:

- Keep your head in line with your spine
- As you breathe out, press your tongue against the roof of your mouth to prevent yourself from over-tightening the jaw and neck muscles
- To prevent straining your neck when rising, don't focus your gaze on your knees; instead focus on something in the distance
- Don't lace your fingers behind your neck when rising; the temptation to pull on the neck for support is hard to resist, instead, use your elbows for balance

Spine relaxer

Sitting cross-legged, stomach held in, bend forward and hold your arms out on the floor in front of you. Hold for the count of ten and then relax.

Back and arms

This may sound rather tricky but it is very relaxing. Again sitting cross-legged on the floor with your back straight, clench your hands behind your back, clasp your fingers together and gently pull on them for a count of ten. Then relax.

Ab tenser

Lie face down on the floor, with your elbows slightly bent so that they are under your shoulders. Making sure the forearms and elbows remain on the floor, raise both head and shoulders very slowly. Hold this position for a count of six, then relax.

Exercising Options

If the concept of donning a leotard and taking up step aerobics at the local gym fills you with horror, or the mere mention of jogging causes an outbreak of athlete's foot, relax – there are plenty of other options! We shall look at some of them on these two pages.

Kick boxing

This activity has become very popular with both men and women. Furthermore it:

✓ Helps lower body fat by toning the muscles
✓ Helps people to work out their stresses and frustrations
✓ Improves power, balance, and overall agility
✓ Increases muscular endurance and strength
✓ Many women say that it enhances their self-confidence
✓ Tones and conditions the upper part of the body

Many local gyms run kick-boxing classes, so why not check them out?

Cycling

The idea of squeezing into a pair of Lycra shorts and hitting the highways on your bike may not fill you with an adrenalin rush but when you consider its health benefits, it is well-worth a second thought.

Cycling is an ideal exercise for toning up muscles, getting out in the fresh air and just popping out to the shops. If you are a little hesitant of what people may say, you could always borrow or hire an indoor cycle or nip along to your local gym to use their

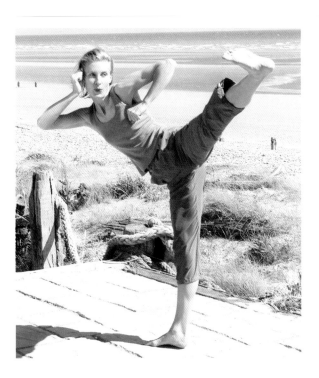

cycling machines. Admittedly, cycling indoors can be a little boring, although you can always wear some earphones and tune in to some music to while away the time spent exercising.

Water aerobics

This is based on normal aerobic exercises, i.e. running, jogging and walking, but instead of it being done on land, the exercises are performed in water, generally at a local swimming pool. It is a perfect form of all-round exercise and, as your confidence grows, so you will find yourself able to move into a deeper section

Take care

If you have any chronic medical conditions or back problems, you should consult your doctor before starting any exercise program.

of the pool. Essentially the idea is to work the muscles against the resistance of the water while maintaining an upright stance throughout the exercise sequence. It is a great way of burning up calories efficiently.

Power walking

How about taking up power walking? Not a gentle saunter around the park but a brisk walk, head and shoulders back, arms swinging, stomach held in and taking long determined strides. Not only will it encourage better posture, but power walking is also ideal for toning up the thighs, arms and legs. The more intense you make it, the more calories you will burn up. And when you are powering along, make sure that you take in deep breaths of fresh air.

Gardening

If you don't feel like doing anything beyond your home patch and you have a garden, then look no further for your daily exercise. Mow the lawn – it's great for toning up the abdominal muscles; how about pruning those high branches – no better exercise for toning the arms and back; or pull up weeds – it is the ideal answer for working on those thighs as you bend and straighten. It also helps to tone up buttocks and arms, and the bonus is that your garden looks good too.

Exercising for new mothers

After giving birth, some women are sometimes devastated to find themselves left with saggy stomach muscles. While other parts of the body slowly get back into shape, the stomach often seems reluctant to return to its former shape. But don't worry – with some gentle exercising, those over-stretched muscles will soon disappear and you will be able to climb into those clinging denims again. But before you put on your training clothes and set yourself an exhausting

schedule to follow, here are a few important rules:

• Check with your doctor or local health visitor about exercising and ask if they have any gentle firming-up exercises that they can recommend. Remember childbirth is a traumatic experience for the body and you cannot expect it to snap back into its previous condition just like that.

• Develop a routine. Wait until the baby is having a nap, or has gone to bed, before you start exercising.

• Make sure that each of your movements is slow and take adequate rest breaks between exercises.

• Warm up and cool down before and after each exercise session by doing a few gentle stretching movements.

• If one day you feel under the weather or it is hot, reduce your routine by half, and make sure that you drink plenty of water to prevent dehydration.

• Simply taking the baby out for a walk is good exercise; remember that a happy contented mother makes for a happy contented baby.

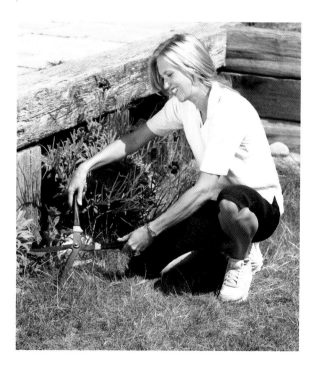

A Good Diet

If you turn green with envy every time you see a young model flaunting her well-toned abdomen, don't imagine that she didn't have to make an effort to achieve it.

Remember, it doesn't matter how much exercise you do, it can never fully compensate for poor eating habits. The only way to eliminate surplus fat is:

✓ To change your eating habits
✓ To increase your level of exercise

By sticking to these two basic rules, you will be well on your way to achieving that perfect stomach.

Nourishing the body

Changing eating habits does not mean that you have to follow a diet and count all your calories. What it does mean is that you should eat healthy nourishing

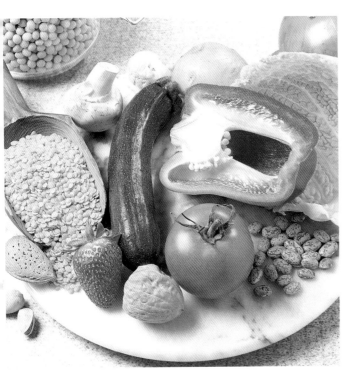

food containing a balance of essential nutrients, which in turn are derived from the following:

Carbohydrates: These provide energy for the body and come in two basic forms. Simple carbohydrates basically comprise sugar and very little else. Complex carbohydrates include starchy foods, such as bread, potatoes, cereal, pasta, rice, etc.

Fats: The number one enemy in terms of a lean body but essential for helping to insulate and protect the organs and nerves. It is found in varying quantities in numerous foods such as butter, cheese, lard, snack-type foods, fatty meat, etc. The basic principle of a healthy diet is to reduce the amount of fat you eat and stick to a low-fat diet. It doesn't mean cutting fat out totally, but rather choosing those foods sensibly and checking on the label for a low-fat alternative.

Proteins: The body breaks down the protein from food into its component parts, called amino acids, which it then uses to build and repair tissue and muscle. Protein is found in foods such as meat, poultry, fish, dairy foods, eggs, beans, lentils and nuts, cheese, yogurt, etc.

Minerals: These are vital to the human body as they help to form bones, strengthen teeth, maintain a healthy immune system, and support the vitamins in their work. Calcium, for instance, is important for helping to build strong bones and teeth.

Vitamins: These substances are vital for good health and the maintenance of various bodily functions. A well-balanced diet containing plenty of fresh foods should be rich in vitamins. .

Each day on the program make sure that you:

Eat three meals a day: breakfast, lunch and dinner. Your daily intake should include:

- 6oz protein food – fish, poultry, cottage cheese, lean meat
- 12oz vegetables
- 12oz fresh fruit
- 6oz bread, cereal, potatoes, rice, pasta
- $3/4$ pint 1 or 2 per cent milk
- $1/4$ pint unsweetened orange, grapefruit or apple juice
- Tea and coffee can be drunk using milk from your quota but try drinking more water instead

Foods that can cause problems

Some people react badly to certain foods that cause bloatedness, gas, and other related digestive disorders. Often it is possible to trace those foods responsible by trial and error and so eliminate them from your diet.

If you suffer from bloatedness, it may well be triggered off by eating one of the foods listed below. If you are unsure, keep a record every time you eat them to monitor whether there are any recurrent symptoms and you can avoid the food in question.

- Alcohol
- Beans
- Bran
- Brussels sprouts
- Cauliflower
- Cheese
- Coffee
- Fizzy drinks
- Garlic
- Onion
- Peas
- Processed foods, i.e. canned meats
- Pulses
- Salt
- Tea

On the other hand, certain foods can counteract that bloatedness, especially when it is related to pre-menstrual syndrome (PMS).

- Celery
- Citrus fruits
- Fish
- Green leafy vegetables
- Meat
- Natural water
- Parsley
- Wholegrains

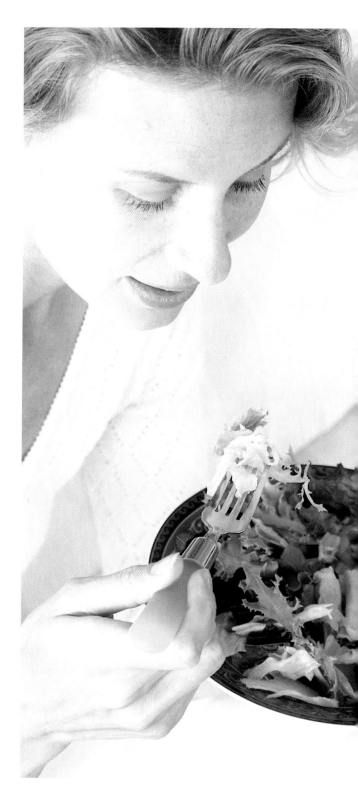

Ban these foods!

If you are really serious about following this program then certain types of food must be banned, unless in very special circumstances they are unavoidable:

Meats

- Black pudding
- Fat or skin from all meat and poultry
- Goose and other fatty meat
- Haggis
- Pâté
- Pork pie
- Salami
- Sausage
- Scotch eggs

Dairy produce

- All cheese, except cottage cheese
- Butter
- Cream
- Dripping
- Egg custard
- Eggs and other related products
- Full-fat milk
- Ice cream
- Lard
- Low-fat spreads containing more than 4 per cent fat and all similar products
- Margarine
- Quiches
- Suet

Other foods

- All fried foods
- Avocados
- Cakes
- Chips
- Chocolate
- Chocolate spread
- Cocoa and related products
- Cookies
- Fudge
- Lemon curd
- Marzipan
- Pastries – sweet and savory
- Peanut butter
- Sauces and dressings which contain cream, whole milk, or eggs
- Sponge desserts

Low-fat food

While you are on this 28-day program, you will have to cut out certain favorite foods, but with such a wide and varied choice remaining for you, that will not seem such a hardship unless you are a veritable slave to cakes and chocolate. All the time you are abstaining, remember the reason that you doing so – a lean, taut abdomen.

There are several ways to help cut back the fat content in your food:

1. When shopping, make sure that you always pay attention to the nutritional contents printed on the side of the packaged food you buy. The two most important details are the total fat and energy content. The energy value on the sides of food packaging will be shown in kilojoules or kilocalories (kcal). The kcal figure tells you the number of calories per 4oz. Ideally select foods containing no more than 0.14oz of fat per 4oz of weight. Don't be tempted by those foods that simply say they are low-fat – always check the label to confirm this for yourself.

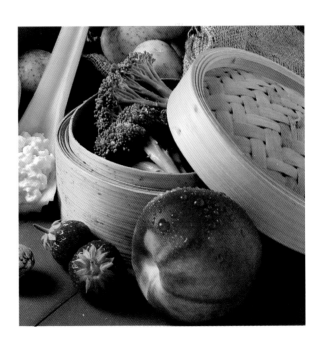

2. Use 1 or 2 per cent milk.

3. Whenever possible, steam, broil or bake food, instead of frying it.

4. Use low-fat yogurt instead of cream or ice cream.

5. Eat cottage cheese instead of full-fat cheese.

6. Add more fish and poultry to your diet.

7. Always trim any visible fat off meat.

8. Simmer ingredients in vegetable stock instead of shallow frying them in lard or butter.

Of course you do need a small amount of fat in your diet but, by following these guidelines, you will ensure that you do not get too much.

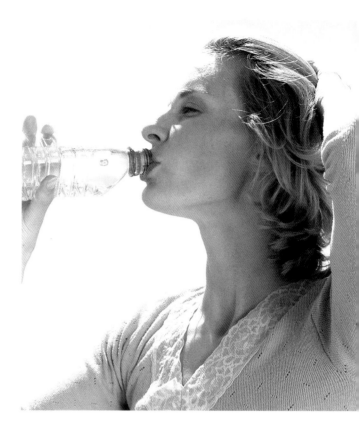

What you can have

It's not all bad news as there are lots of tempting and tasty foods that you can enjoy throughout the program and lots of delicious menus you can experiment with. For example:

Bread: The staff of life and fine to eat providing it is wholemeal.

Cottage cheese: You don't have to stick with the plain variety, there are lots of differently flavored low-fat ones that make a refreshing addition to a salad. Try some spread on crispbread for a quick lunchtime snack or, if you are having friends around, add a handful of herbs and garlic to plain cottage cheese as it makes a tasty dip .

Gravy: If you cannot face a meal without gravy, just ensure that you make it using gravy powder and not the meat juices.

Pasta and rice: Nutritious and satisfying – whenever possible stick to the wholemeal varieties.

Vegetables: You can choose whatever you like, even potatoes, but just make sure they are steamed or boiled rather than fried and don't add butter! Eaten raw, carrots, celery, and pea pods are all very tasty.

Sauces: To add some extra flavour to a slice of bread or to a salad, to pour over fish or pep up a pasta dish, you can have a virtually free range with the following:

- Brown, chilli, horseradish, mint, Worcester sauces
- Fat-free salad dressings
- Lemon juice
- Marmite
- Mustard
- Oil-free vinaigrette dressing
- Soy sauce
- Vinegar

Drinks: Aim to drink at least five or six large glasses of water each day, especially during the summer months. Tea and coffee are fine providing any milk is deducted from your daily quota and, if possible, try drinking it without adding sugar. It's far healthier. Diet drinks are fine, but natural water is even better and the occasional weekend glass of wine is allowed.

A New Eating Regime

The main principle to remember when following this eating plan is that you must maximize your fat loss by adopting a low-fat diet and taking plenty of exercise.

The main reason why people don't succeed when following an eating regime is that they:
- are impatient and expect to see results immediately
- are not sufficiently motivated
- don't eat enough at the prescribed mealtimes
- don't understand their bodies' needs
- eat too little overall
- exercise on an empty stomach

Here are some suggestions for you to select from – there is lots of variety. To make it easier why not decide every day on the meals for the following day and, whenever possible, prepare them before going to bed. In that way you will not have to worry about what to eat as soon as you get up.

Breakfast suggestions

Each of the following may be served with some of the milk from the daily allowance:
- $1/5$ cup muesli, 1 teaspoon sugar, 1 sliced banana
- 1 cup All-Bran with 1 teaspoon sugar, 1 chopped apple
- 2 cups cornflakes with 1 teaspoon sugar, 1 cup strawberries
- 2 Weetabix with 1 teaspoon sugar, 1 sliced banana
- To make your own muesli, place $1/6$ cup porridge oats, 6 golden raisins, 1 teaspoon clear honey, $1/2$ cup 1 per cent milk and 5fl oz natural yogurt in a bowl, cover and place it in the refrigerator to chill until morning.

Fruity breakfasts
- 1 grapefruit and 2 small pots of low-fat yogurt

- 1 cup stewed fruit cooked without sugar and topped with 1 small carton of low-fat yogurt
- 11oz can grapefruit segments in natural juice
- 5 canned prunes in natural juice and 1 small low-fat natural yogurt
- Slice of melon topped with 4oz grapes and 1 small low-fat yogurt
- Chop up one apple, peel and slice a banana and an orange, then mix them together with a handful of grapes in a bowl.

Hot options
- 2 slices wholemeal bread topped with 3 teaspoons marmalade or honey
- 1 whole muffin and 1 apple
- 1 small poached egg served on 1 slice wholemeal toast spread with Marmite and $1/2$ fresh grapefruit

Lunchtime ideas

If midday is a hectic time for you, slow down and take stock. Have a salad one day, a jacket potato with a favorite topping the next, a sandwich the following day and keep ringing the changes to add variety to your midday meal.

- For an apple and carrot salad, sprinkle the juice of half a lemon juice over 3 sliced apples to prevent them discoloring. Mix 1lb of grated carrots 3 tablespoons golden raisins, 1 tablespoon sunflower seeds and 2 tablespoons cashew nuts in the juice with the apples. Tear half an iceberg lettuce into strips and put in a bowl, add the carrot and apple mixture and then blend into the vinaigrette dressing (recipe follows).

• For an oil-free vinaigrette, mix 3 tablespoons white wine vinegar, 1 tablespoon lemon juice, $1^1/_2$ teaspoons black pepper, $^1/_2$ teaspoon salt, 1 teaspoon sugar, $^1/_2$ teaspoon French mustard, and a handful of chopped assorted herbs together. Taste and add more salt or sugar as required. The dressing will keep in the refrigerator for up to three days.

• For a tasty raw beet salad, mix together 2 stalks finely chopped celery, 1 cup peeled and grated raw beet and 2 large dessert apples, cored and chopped and grated carrot to taste. Add enough oil-free vinaigrette dressing to moisten the salad.

• Rice salad is great at lunchtime. Chop up a chunk of cucumber, a tomato, and a green bell pepper very finely. Put them into a bowl. Add $^1/_4$ cup boiled brown rice, $^1/_4$ cup cooked sweetcorn and $^1/_4$ cup cooked peas. Finally add a dash of soy sauce, a sprinkling of black pepper, and a pinch of salt.

• This recipe for stuffed tomatoes serves two. Using a sharp knife cut off the tops of 2 large, firm tomatoes and scoop out the seeds. Open and drain the juice from a small can of sweetcorn and the brine from a small can of tuna fish before transferring them into a bowl. Add 2 tablespoons low-calorie mayonnaise, stir the mixture, and spoon it back into the tomatoes.

Dinner suggestions

• Fish is easily digestible, nutritious, and very versatile. Preheat the oven to 340°F. Grate the rind from half a lemon and season two pieces of plaice with lemon rind, salt, and pepper. Roll up and secure each fillet with a cocktail stick. Place the fillets in a casserole dish, sprinkle with assorted chopped fresh herbs, and cover with any remaining grated rind plus two teaspoons of lemon juice. Cover with a lid. Bake for 40-50 minutes. When the fish is completely white and flakes easily, lift it out and transfer it to a warmed serving dish. Serve with a green salad.

• Chicken stir-fry makes a quick supper dish. Heat 1 tablespoon of sunflower oil or olive oil in a non-stick skillet and partly cook 4oz sliced chicken breast until it changes color. Add 1 medium tin beansprouts, 3 stalks finely sliced celery, 1 Spanish onion, peeled and sliced, and 3oz mushrooms, washed and sliced, a little at a time until all the ingredients are lightly cooked. Serve with $^3/_4$ cup boiled brown rice.

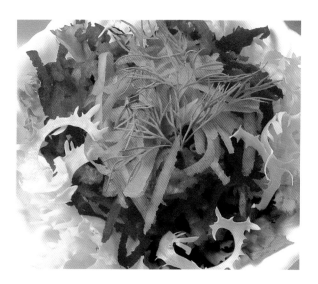

Delicious desserts

• Baked apples. Preheat the oven to 350°F. Cut a ring in the peel around the middle of a large cooking apple and remove the core. Stuff the core with $^1/_2$ tablespoon finely chopped Brazil nuts, 1 tablespoon sultanas and $^1/_2$ teaspoon each of ground cinnamon and ground coriander, place in an ovenproof dish and bake for 35 minutes. Delicious served with low-fat yogurt.

• For a fruit fool, put 2 punnets strawberries, 2 cartons low-fat yogurt, 1 teaspoon honey, and 1 teaspoon natural vanilla essence into a liquidizer and blend until smooth. Serve in a tall glass, sprinkled with flaked almonds or chopped Brazil nuts.

Daily Treatments

Whether you want a flatter stomach to make you feel better, to hold your posture better or
to give you more self-confidence, the aim of this program is to show you how
it can be done with the minimum of pain.

However, there are certain things that you should do each day.

Stretch

Greet each day with an early morning stretch either in bed or first thing when you get up. Stress, watching too much TV, even lying in bed for up to eight hours can all cause muscular aches and pains to develop. Inactivity can ultimately lead to a build-up of lactic acid in the muscles resulting in pain and stiffness. That is why the daily routine of stretching the arms and body is invaluable.

Energy shower

There is nothing quite like an early morning energy shower to kick-start the body into

Make sure that each day you:
- Have a morning stretch
- Take a daily energy shower
- Start the day with a glass of water with a squeeze of lemon or lime juice
- Focus on an inspiring thought appropriate to each day
- Spend 30 minutes exercising
- Include some stomach exercises
- Do 10-15 mini sit-ups each day
- Spend five minutes practicing quality breathing
- Each day pamper yourself in some special way

action, so try each morning to jump into the shower and, if you are feeling brave enough, when you are ready to come out, turn the cold faucet full on for several minutes.

After showering, stimulate your body and boost the circulation by slapping your skin all over. Using the flats of your hands slap from toes to hip, wrist to shoulder and all over your chest, shoulders and torso before rubbing yourself dry with a towel.

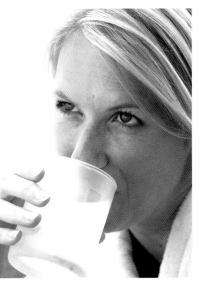

Wake-up drink

Don't forget to start the day with a glass of hot water with an added squeeze of lemon or lime to cleanse your mouth and put a zing in your step.

Exercise

The various types of exercise recommended for toning and strengthening the abdominal area were discussed on pages 12-13. Don't forget that they form a critical part of the program and so should be included every day, even if you don't always feel in the mood. Try to build up the number you can manage gradually day by day.

Inspiring thoughts

When was the last time you seriously thought about yourself and your life? Last week? Last month? Perhaps you can't even remember the last time. Why not make a determined effort throughout this program to allow yourself some quality time to think about your future and what you would like to achieve? It could be something as wacky as doing a bungee jump, or perhaps you would like to start a business of your own, or spend a weekend at a health farm. All of these things are attainable – none need remain a pipe dream. We all need goals in life to aim at, and so why not allow yourself 10 minutes each day to sit down and write how you feel and to record something that you would like to do in the future. It doesn't matter if it sounds weird or bizarre. If that's how you feel, write it down in your diary as an inspiring thought for the day.

Deep breathing

There is nothing quite as invigorating or refreshing as five minutes of deep steady breathing. It blows away those cobwebs and is also an excellent way to de-stress yourself.

1. Sit in a quiet room.
2. If you are wearing a skirt or pants, undo the waistband so there is plenty of room for you to expand your stomach.
3. Close your eyes, now slowly breathe in through your nose and hold that breath for a count of five. Then, to another count of five, slowly exhale through your mouth.
4. Repeat several times until the 5 minutes are up.

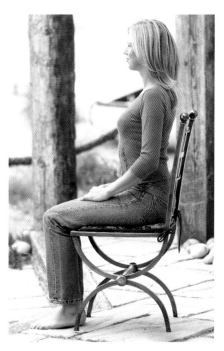

Pamper yourself

And why not? You deserve it; you're a good person, so go out and treat yourself to the biggest, brightest bunch of flowers you can find, book yourself in for a hair appointment, spend one afternoon sifting through your old collections of books and records, or clear out your closet. Whatever takes your fancy, just make sure you allow time for yourself each day.

Good posture

Good posture is achievable. It will not only make you feel better but you will look smarter too.

Here are some simple steps to help you to improve your posture:

1. When walking, make a conscious effort to keep your backbone straight and hold your shoulders back. Pull in your stomach and buttocks and tuck in your chin.
2. When seated, sit up straight and do not cross your legs.
3. If working at a desk choose a seat in which you are comfortable and which is at the correct position for your desk. The seat should be high enough to allow your thighs to rest horizontally on the seat.
4. Wear sensible low-heeled shoes. Keep high ones for the occasional night out. Shoes with low heels put far less strain on your back than stiletto heels.
5. Practice walking around the house with a heavy book balanced on your head, as though you were at a deportment class. The aim is to reach the other end of the room with the book still on your head

Maintaining The Program

Trying to change is never easy and there are bound to be occasions during the 28 days when you think "Why bother? What is the point of it all?" When you have one of those days, sit down and spend a little longer on finding an inspiring thought to lift your spirits.

Remind yourself that you are doing the program because you want to wear a cropped top again on your vacation, you want to feel more confident in how you look, you want get rid of that surplus bulge around your midriff which has been reluctant to move since you had your last child.

The 28 day plan is not meant to be an ordeal. Yes, you will have to be prepared for a little hard work at times, but it should not be something you dread doing. It is important that you set aside an hour or so each day for a bit of personal TLC. On these pages, I suggest various ideas for making you feel good about yourself.

Flower power

Studies carried out in America have shown that if you surround yourself with flowers, they can trigger off feelings of happiness, soothe away anxieties, and improve your quality of life. So if Mr Right has not bought you a bunch recently, take the initiative and buy yourself some.

Reading

Choose a really good novel and curl up one afternoon for a couple of hours to read it. If it makes you cry, so much the better – everyone needs a good cry now and then. It can help to relieve stress.

Hand pampering

If your hands are feeling slightly dry and could do with some pampering, mix a teaspoon of honey with two teaspoons of olive oil and massage it into your hands after washing them in warm soapy water and

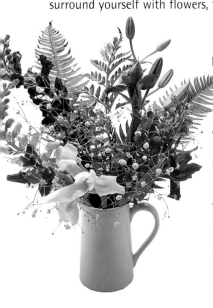

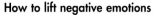

How to lift negative emotions
- Keep a record of those negative thoughts. Write them down in a diary and then start to challenge them by putting positive messages alongside. "I don't feel that I'm looking any better" may be a negative message, "but you are doing a lot more than before and are much fitter" could be the positive reply.
- If you have times when you feel anxious or stressed out, stop and think about happy occasions and try to remember how they felt.
- Ignore negative thoughts whenever they worm their way into your mind. After all, millions of thoughts pass through our minds each day; thoughts can't harm you.
- Set yourself a challenge – take up a new sport and aspire to a certain level of proficiency. By achieving this, you will feel much more confident of your abilities.

drying them gently. Pop a pair of cotton gloves on and go to bed wearing the gloves, allowing the oil to soak in overnight In the morning wash your hands in warm soapy water. They will feel soft and clean.

Surf the internet

Have you often wished that you could surf the net, but you are frustrated because you don't know the first thing about it? Well, now's the time to change all that! If you have a computer and modem at home, there is no time like the present to learn a new skill. There are lots of books in the library telling you how to get online, and some local colleges run short introductory courses on the subject. Once you have a basic understanding, you will find that the internet opens up a whole new world to you.

Thinking positive

You may well face days during the program when you are plagued by negative thoughts, but hidden beneath those dull feelings are positive emotions lying in wait. So work hard each day to bring them to the fore. When you feel good about yourself, you can begin to understand and accept the type of person you are and not punish yourself mentally for any shortcomings or imperfections. We are all human, after all. Experts have found that people who are positive and optimistic enjoy long-term good health.

Minty bath

If you are looking for a bath with a difference then try this one. You need:
- 1 cup chopped fresh mint
- 1 cup chopped bay leaves
- 1 teaspoon coconut oil
- 1 teaspoon almond extract

Add all the ingredients into a bowl and stir well. Cut a piece of cheesecloth or similar material into a large square and tie it into a pouch. Drop the ingredients into the middle of the square and tie the ends together. When drawing the hot water for a bath, dip the pouch into the flowing water and allow the herbs time to infuse. Once the water has cooled down to a comfortable temperature, step into the bathtub, and relax for 30 minutes.

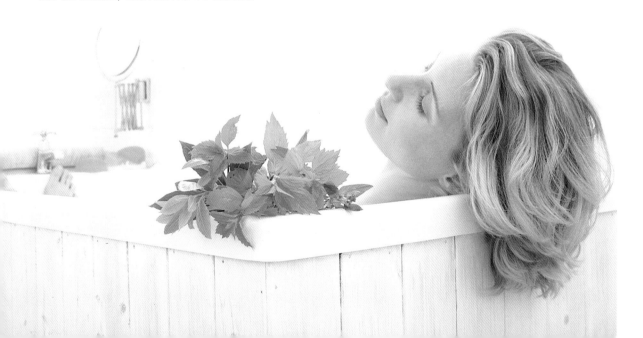

Flat Stomach: Days 1–7

You've done all the preparatory work and now can look forward to a 28-day program that should leave you feeling invigorated and rejuvenated.

Whether you are a working woman or a busy mother at home, the next 28 days should witness some of the biggest changes that you will ever make to your life...so be prepared! Draw up a chart (see page 31) and stick it on your refridgerator or kitchen wall so that you will remember exactly what you must include on each day of your program.

Keep a diary and record in it your everyday thoughts. Even if you have had a rotten day, write it down and then try to understand why it was such a bad day. At the end of each day summarize how you feel. Naturally on some days you will find more to write about than on others, but it will help to keep you motivated if you keep this diary and refer to it for encouragement when you have down days.

One good tip to keep you motivated is to take a skirt out of your closet, one that is slightly too cozy around the waist, and call it "the flabby skirt." Make a record of your measurements on the first day of your program and pin it on to the waistband of the skirt. Whenever you have moments of self-doubt, remind yourself of how nice it would be to wear that skirt without it pinching. That ambition is achievable.

Here is a typical plan for day 1, but of course times and the order in which activities are performed may differ, according to your individual lifestyle.

7.00am Early morning stretch – spend 10 minutes stretching and flexing those tired, stiff muscles. Open your bedroom window and let in some fresh air before you begin.

7.15am Refresh your mouth and body with a glass of hot water to which a squeeze of fresh lemon juice has been added.

8.00am Have an energy shower.

8.45am Time for breakfast. Why not just eat fruit this morning?

9.30am Go for a brisk 30-minute power walk.

11.00am Have a glass of water and spend five minutes on quality breathing.

1.00pm Lunch. Try a beet salad.

2.15pm Time to do some sit-ups. Just aim to do ten today and remember to include the warm-up and cooling-down exercises too. Afterward relax and read a book with a cup of herbal tea.

4.00pm Find a quiet place, sit down and think about some goal that you would like to achieve within the next few years. Write it down on paper and imagine how it can be attained.

6.00pm Prepare dinner, perhaps some fish this evening. Enjoy a piece of fruit for dessert.

7.00pm Why not indulge in a minty bath and subtly illuminate the bathroom with candles?

8.00pm End the first day by giving your nails a manicure. Then climb into bed with a good book and read for a while until drowsiness overtakes you.

Don't forget: As you complete each activity, tick it off on your chart and before you go to sleep remember to record in your diary how you felt, noting down both the good and the bad points.

Remainder of the week

The remainder of week 1 should follow more or less the same pattern but add some different foods and try different exercises to keep things fresh. Don't try increasing the sit-ups or stomach exercises until the latter part of the week.

Measurements chart

As you change your routine to include more exercise and reform your eating habits, you will find that you are not only achieving a flatter stomach but you will have toned up muscles all over your body to give you a slimmer look and lots more energy!

You can record your measurements each week using this simple chart.

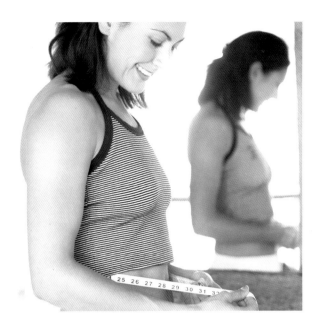

	Week 1	Week 2	Week 3	Week 4
Date				
Weight				
Bust				
Waist				
Hips				

Exercise diary

It is a good idea to keep an exercise diary like the example below. Make a note of the activities you have undertaken and how you felt afterward and you will soon begin to see clear signs of improvement in stamina and fitness.

Fill it in at the end of each day and by the end of the program you will see how much more you are able to do than at the beginning.

Week 1	Exercise	Length of time/distance	Comments
April 1st	Walking	12 minutes/half a mile	Shattered
April 2nd	Walking	10 minutes/half a mile	Breathless
	Sit ups	20 minutes	Exhausted, felt super
April 3rd	Swimming	40 minutes/8 lengths	Exhilarated but tired

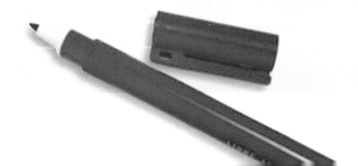

Flat Stomach: Days 8–14

One week down, only three to go! By now certain routines should be established and you should be used to the program.

But remember, no slacking! And don't start eating foods that are banned!

7.00am Early morning stretch – spend 10 minutes stretching and flexing those tired muscles. Open your bedroom window and let in some fresh air before you begin.

7.15am Refresh your mouth and body with a glass of hot water to which a squeeze of lime or lemon juice has been added.

8.00am Take an energy shower or perhaps try having a bath this week doing exactly the same as when showering i.e. turning the cold faucet on full and splashing the cool water over your body before getting out.

8.45am Time for breakfast. Muesli today!

9.30am Spend time doing your stomach exercises. Then have a glass of water; you will almost certainly need it after that workout.

11.00am Perhaps you have had an inspiring idea that you would like to pursue. You could try writing some poetry or a story.

1.00pm Lunch. If you are meeting friends for lunch, then make sure that you choose a low-fat dish, possibly a baked potato or a sandwich containing low-fat ingredients. Remember, read the labels if you

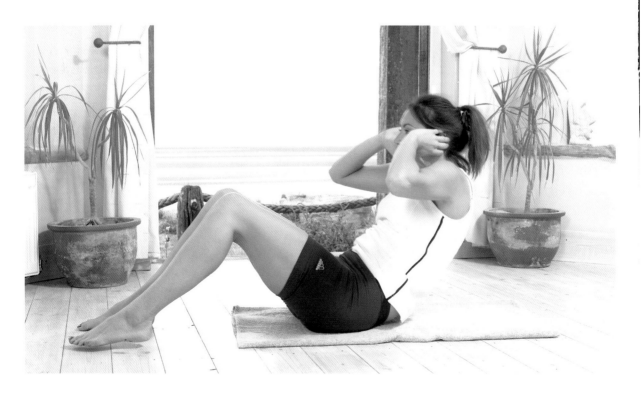

De-stress yourself

When things are getting on top of you and you dread going to bed in case worries and concerns worm their way into your subconscious mind, it is time for action. This is how to relax totally.

• Lie or sit down, whichever feels more comfortable.

• Close your eyes and imagine a favorite room; it could be any room, anywhere. Say to yourself "Nothing else matters."

• Concentrate on all the objects in that room that make it so special to you, such as the drapes or the pictures hanging on the walls.

• Now eradicate each and every one of those images one by one until there is nothing at all left. The room is empty.

• Keep this image in your mind for a few moments and while you do so luxuriate in the sensation of total peace and tranquillity. You have never felt so totally relaxed and your mind is free of unwanted thoughts.

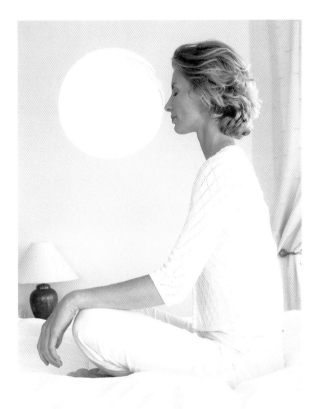

are buying pre-packed products. Complement the food with a glass of fresh juice.

2.15pm If you feel guilty at having taken longer than normal over lunch, why not do some power walking for 30 minutes?

4.00pm Get your exercise gear on again for some mini sit-ups. By now you may be in a position to increase the number slightly, but don't rush. Afterward make sure you cool down and have a glass or two of water to replenish any lost fluids.

6.00pm Prepare dinner. Tonight I suggest a chicken meal with rice.

7.00pm Practice some deep breathing and then pamper yourself – do a crossword, listen to some music, enjoy anything that you find relaxing for an hour or two.

8.00pm It has been a busy day, so have an early night! If you have trouble getting off to sleep or are plagued by negative thoughts, try the de-stressing routine described below.

Don't forget: As you complete each activity, tick it off on your chart and before you go to sleep remember to record in your diary how you felt, noting down both the good and the bad points.

Remainder of the week

The rest of week 2 should follow more or less the same basic routine, but don't let boredom set in. Set yourself little targets. You might see if there are any local aerobic classes held nearby which you could join. Group activities give you a chance to meet other people and help to keep you motivated. Better still, if your place of work has a gym, why not spend part of your lunchtime working out?

Flat Stomach: Days 15–21

You will by now have established a routine and perhaps made some changes to personalize the program to suit your lifestyle.

So are you ready for week 3? You are now half-way through the program and are probably getting used to the new lifestyle.

7.00am Early morning stretch – spend 10 minutes stretching and flexing those tired muscles. Open your bedroom window and let in some fresh air before you begin.

7.15am Refresh your mouth and body with a glass of hot water to which a squeeze of lemon juice has been added.

8.00am Have an energy shower.

8.45am Time for breakfast. Have a muffin with some Marmite on it.

9.30am Why not try another exercise activity this week; you might take up cycling or try some water aerobics. Or you could do some gardening – all the bending is an excellent way of exercising your stomach. Don't forget the warm-up routine beforehand.

11.00am Time to stop for a cup of water and a few minutes' rest. If it's a nice day, you could do some quality breathing outside sitting in a chair in the sunshine.

1.00pm Lunch. If you have expended energy gardening, you will be feeling pretty hungry so you might prepare yourself a tuna salad with a small low-fat yogurt to follow.

2.15pm Spend about 15 minutes doing mini sit-ups. By now you should easily be able to manage at least 40 sit-ups without adverse effects.

4.00pm By the third week you should have begun to notice that your stomach muscles are looking slightly more toned and you should generally be feeling healthier. You deserve a treat, so go and buy yourself a bunch of flowers.

6.00pm Dinner. A vegetable and chicken stir-fry followed by baked apples is delicious. Try to get someone else to wash the dishes and sit down for a while to watch the TV or catch up on that book you've almost finished.

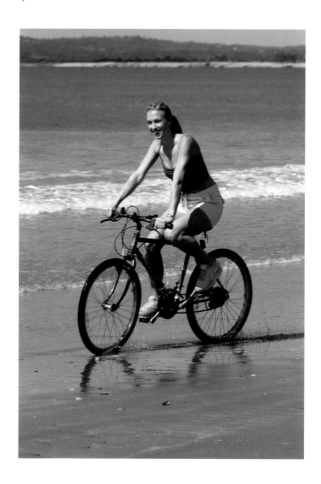

Warm-up gardening exercises

It's amazing how strenuous gardening can be and how much strain it puts on certain parts of the body, especially the back and legs. Make sure before you get down to weeding or mowing the lawn that you do some warm-up exercises beforehand.

1. You will need a good overall stretch. With your hands above your head, stretch as far as you are able sideways, hold for a count of 15, and then stretch to the opposite side, again holding the pose for a count of 15. Relax.

2. The legs, especially the hamstrings, can take some punishment, so you need to stretch them thoroughly. Stand upright and place your hands on one leg just above the knee. Gently lean forward and, making sure the other leg remains straight, bend down slowly. You should feel the stretch in the back of your thigh. Hold for a count of 8, then do the same with the other leg.

3. When you've finished gardening, lie on the floor face-down, slowly lift your upper body a little, and stretch backward. This is the perfect exercise to counteract the strain that your spine has been subjected to after all the forward bending that gardening requires.

7.00pm If, toward the middle of the third week, you are beginning to feel anxious and worried that you won't reach your target, that you're having a rotten day and nothing is going right, your stomach still looks flabby, and you've eaten a forbidden chocolate bar, take time out to de-stress (see pages 26–27).

8.00pm Have an early night – tomorrow will be better!

Don't forget: As you complete each activity, tick it off on your chart and before you go to sleep remember to record in your diary how you felt, noting down both the good and the bad points.

Remainder of the week

Keep up with the routine even if you don't feel like doing it some days. If you hit a bad patch and feel really down in the dumps, do something positive – go out and buy yourself a treat, ask a friend around, or, if you are a mother, take the kids swimming after school. Jump into the water too – the kids will love it and there's no better way of teaching youngsters how much fun exercising can be.

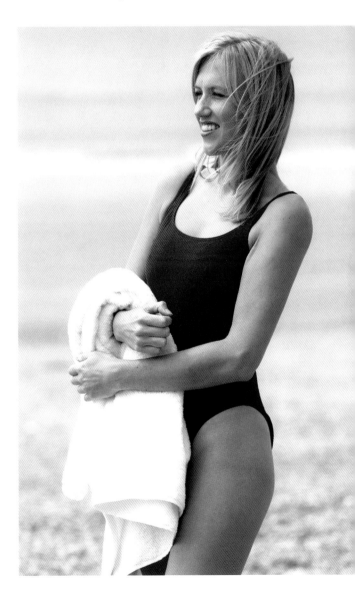

Flat Stomach: Days 22–28

This is it! You are nearing the end of your 28-day Flat Stomach program and you have survived. You should begin to feel more energetic now, largely on account of a healthier diet combined with regular exercise and relaxation.

So don't give up now. Why throw away all your hard-won gains?

7.00am Early morning stretch – spend 10 minutes stretching and flexing those tired muscles. Open your bedroom window and let in some fresh air before you begin.

7.15am Refresh your mouth and body with a glass of hot water to which a squeeze of lime juice has been added.

8.00am Have an energy shower.

8.45am Time for breakfast. Why not choose something hot for a change?

9.30am Time for some stomach workouts. They should be no problem by now.

11.00am Have a cup of herbal tea before popping out to the shops.

1.00pm Lunch. If a friend is coming around, you might prepare some healthy sandwiches.

2.15pm Go out for a cycle ride. Make sure you plan a route that takes you along roads that are not too busy. If you feel embarrassed to be seen cycling around the neighborhood, you can always pack the bike into your car and drive somewhere quiet for a 30-minute cycle. Remember don't go too far from the car; you need to conserve enough energy to get back

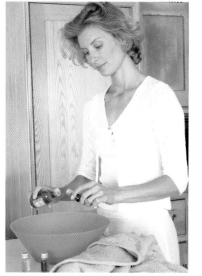

to it at the end of the ride.

4.00pm If you feel exhausted after the cycle ride, do some quality breathing and then recharge your batteries with a glass of freshly squeezed orange juice.

6.00pm Prepare a special meal for family or friends, perhaps pasta with salad. And because it is nearly the end of your program, you can treat yourself to a glass of wine.

7.00pm Sit down and round off your "inspiring thought" plan. Leave it for a few days and then go back and review it in the light of the progress you have made over the four-week period.

8.00pm Enjoy a relaxing bath with some favorite essential oils and then have an early night to recover from the exertions of the day.

Don't forget: As you complete each activity, tick it off on your chart and before you go to sleep remember to record in your diary how you felt, noting down both the good and the bad points.

Remainder of the week

Keep up with the routine right through to the very last day. On the final day why not celebrate, and treat yourself to some new exercise clothes? If you are feeling really good, from now on exercise will become part of your daily life.

Activity Record Chart
Record your activities every day using this table

DAILY ACTIVITIES	1	2	3	4	5	6	7	8	9	10	11	12	13	14	15	16	17	18	19	20	21	22	23	24	25	26	27	28
Morning stretch																												
Glass of hot water and lemon or lime juice																												
Shower/bath																												
Breakfast																												
Lunch																												
Dinner																												
Fresh vegetables																												
Fresh fruit																												
Protein food																												
3/4 pint 1 or 2 per cent milk																												
3 pints water																												
10 mins inspiring thought																												
10 mins stomach exercises																												
30 mins exercise																												
10–15 mins sit-ups																												
Pampering																												
5 mins quality breathing																												

Congratulations!

Provided you have followed the program properly and done the exercises as recommended, and not fallen off the wagon and allowed yourself too many "treats", your hard work should now have paid off and you will be the proud owner of a well-toned flat stomach.

Don't worry if you still have a little way to go to achieve that dream washboard abdomen – remember that everyone's metabolism is different and you have done really well to get this far.

You might now want to jump onto the scales to find out exactly how much weight you have lost. Then try on that flabby skirt that you put to one side and check whether there is now plenty of room for maneuver. If you feel happy with the way you look, then you can allow yourself to loosen up a little and relax your eating regime. But be careful! It's very easy to return to old habits.

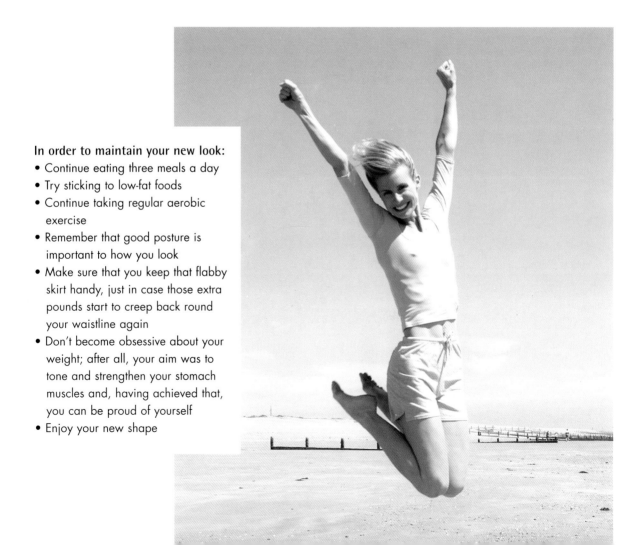

In order to maintain your new look:
- Continue eating three meals a day
- Try sticking to low-fat foods
- Continue taking regular aerobic exercise
- Remember that good posture is important to how you look
- Make sure that you keep that flabby skirt handy, just in case those extra pounds start to creep back round your waistline again
- Don't become obsessive about your weight; after all, your aim was to tone and strengthen your stomach muscles and, having achieved that, you can be proud of yourself
- Enjoy your new shape